THE TRAIL WESTWARD

Westerns for Seniors

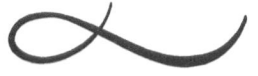

seniorality

The Trail Westward -
Sam Suncroft
Copyright © 2024
Seniorality / Everbreeze Media Oy

This is a work of fiction. Names and characters are the product of the author's imagination and any resemblance to actual persons, living or dead, is entirely coincidental.

Set in EB Garamond

1. Frontier Dreams

Colt Evans guided his horse through the narrow, mud-caked streets of a small frontier town, his sharp eyes scanning each face and shadow as he passed. The town was loud and busy, the sounds of hammers against wood and the laughter of rowdy settlers filling the air. Dust from the trail still clung to his boots, his coat, even his beard— a thin layer that seemed to blend him with the land he knew so well. It had been weeks since he last saw a real town, longer since he'd exchanged more than a few words with anyone. His life on the edge of the wild, where the line between life and death was thin, had hardened him. But today, he had a purpose that went beyond survival.

Colt's gaze sharpened as he glanced toward a makeshift tent set up by the edge of town. A sign, barely clinging to its nail, read: "Pioneer Caravan

Meeting - New Recruits Welcome." Just under that, in smaller letters, someone had scrawled, "Heading West". His lips set in a thin line. Colt didn't care much for company, especially company that involved families and children, all clinging to dreams of the new frontier. But this caravan was different. Somewhere in the midst of hopeful pioneers was the man responsible for his mentor's death. And Colt was ready to find him.

He adjusted his hat and nudged his horse toward the tent, the sounds of conversation and laughter growing louder. As he tied his horse to a nearby post, a movement caught his eye—a woman, standing near the tent's entrance, her shoulders square and her chin held high. She was dressed in a plain dress, practical boots, and a hat that looked like it had weathered a few storms of its own. Her hair, a deep auburn, glinted in the afternoon sun, escaping in loose tendrils from beneath her hat. She looked out over the crowd with an expression that was equal parts determination and apprehension.

Colt took a moment to watch her. Something about her seemed out of place, like she didn't quite belong among the other settlers. While the others chatted and joked, she stood alone, keeping a wary distance. Her eyes, a bright green that seemed almost unnatural against the dust and grit of the town, scanned the crowd with a cautious intensity. She noticed him looking and met his gaze, her mouth tightening into a line before she turned her attention back to the crowd.

With a quiet grunt, Colt approached the tent, sliding past a few eager families who seemed to be spilling out of the tent's flaps. The sounds inside grew louder as he stepped into the packed space. Men were haggling over supplies, mothers were clutching their children close, and the caravan leader—a burly man with graying hair and a booming voice—was outlining the journey's expected challenges to a group of wide-eyed pioneers.

"Listen up, folks," the leader said. "We're headin' west. That means hard trails, unpredictable weather, and more than a few dangers. If you ain't prepared for that, I suggest you turn back now."

Colt narrowed his eyes, studying the man's face. This was Adam Blackthorn, a guide with a reputation for taking people to the frontier and, occasionally, losing a few along the way. It was rumored that he cared more about his pay than the lives he led westward. And judging by his expression—set and cold, with the hint of a smirk—Colt didn't doubt it. Standing beside him was a figure Colt recognized instantly: Judd Barrett, Blackthorn's enforcer, a brute of a man with a sour disposition and a sneer that could send a chill down anyone's spine.

As he considered his next move, a soft voice caught his attention. "Is this your first time heading west?"

Colt turned and found himself looking into those green eyes he'd noticed earlier. Up close, they were even brighter, with a sharpness that belied her calm tone. He cleared his throat, tipping his hat slightly. "I've been through the territory a time or two," he replied. "But I'm no settler."

Her gaze lingered on him, as though weighing the truth in his words. "I didn't figure you for one," she said. "But then, why join a caravan?"

Colt's jaw tightened as he looked back at Blackthorn and Barrett. "Sometimes a man's got business to settle."

She gave him a look that hinted she understood more than he'd expected. "So do I," she replied, her voice barely a whisper.

Before he could ask her meaning, Blackthorn's voice boomed again. "Any more questions? No? Good. If you're stayin', we leave at dawn. Meet at the edge of town. Bring only what you need, and remember, the trail's no place for the faint-hearted."

As the crowd began to disperse, Colt caught the woman's arm gently, halting her. She looked down at his hand, then back up at him, her expression curious. "What's your name?" he asked.

"Lily Harlow," she answered, her voice steady. She looked him up and down, her eyes sharp, almost as though sizing him up. "And yours?"

"Colt Evans."

A flicker of recognition crossed her face. "I've heard that name. Aren't you a trapper?"

"I am," he said simply. "And you don't seem like the type to join a wagon train."

She offered him a faint smile. "Funny, I could say the same about you."

He almost smiled back. Almost. "Maybe you could."

They stood there in silence for a moment, two strangers amidst the dust and chatter of the caravan crowd. Finally, Colt released her arm, nodding as he took a step back. "Guess I'll see you on the trail."

Lily held his gaze, her eyes reflecting something he couldn't quite place—a mix of resolve and sadness. "Guess you will," she said.

As she turned to walk away, Colt's mind whirled with questions. What kind of business could a woman like her have on such a dangerous trail? And why was she here alone?

But he knew better than to pry. They all had their reasons for going west, their pasts trailing behind them like shadows. He watched her disappear into the crowd, her figure blending with the other pioneers until she was nothing more than another face, another secret.

Colt adjusted his hat, took a deep breath, and scanned the crowd once more, his gaze settling on Adam Blackthorn and Judd Barrett as they packed up the tent. For the first time in months, Colt felt something close to hope. He didn't know how long the journey would take, or what dangers lay ahead, but he knew one thing: the answers he'd been searching for lay somewhere on that trail.

2. Caravan of Hope

The dawn broke soft and gray over the frontier town, casting long shadows across the hastily packed wagons lining up at the edge of town. Colt Evans stood near his horse, watching the scene unfold with a quiet intensity. The caravan was bigger than he'd expected, at least twenty wagons, each loaded with supplies, livestock, and wide-eyed settlers eager to carve out a new life. Some were still making last-minute adjustments, tying down barrels of provisions and checking the wheels. Others stood off to the side, huddled together, sharing nervous whispers.

As Colt took it all in, he felt a presence behind him. Turning, he found himself face-to-face with Judd Barrett. The enforcer's scowl was as unwelcoming as Colt had imagined, and his large frame blocked out the morning sun, casting a shadow over Colt's view.

"You're the trapper, huh?" Judd's voice was low, his tone thick with disdain.

Colt met his gaze without flinching. "That's right. Name's Colt Evans."

Judd looked him up and down, his expression barely hiding his contempt. "Seems a little odd for a trapper to be tagging along with a bunch of settlers. What's your game?"

Colt's lips tightened into a thin smile. "Maybe I'm just lookin' for a change of scenery. Same as anyone else."

Judd's eyes narrowed, and he took a step closer, his broad shoulders tense. "Listen here, Evans. I don't care what brought you here, but I don't take kindly to strangers poking their noses where they don't belong. I keep order in this caravan, and I don't need some loner out here stirring up trouble."

Colt didn't flinch. He was used to men like Judd—bullies who relied on their size and force to intimidate others. But Colt had survived harsher terrain and deadlier predators than this enforcer. "I'm not here to make trouble," Colt replied evenly. "But I don't take orders from men like you, either."

A tense silence settled between them, and for a moment, Colt thought Judd might throw a punch. Instead, the enforcer leaned in close, his voice a menacing growl. "You'll do well to remember that Adam Blackthorn's the one in charge here, not you. Stick to whatever fool's errand you're on and stay out of our way."

With that, Judd turned and stomped off, his boots kicking up small clouds of dust. Colt watched him go, feeling the familiar burn of frustration in his chest. This wasn't the first time he'd faced opposition, but Judd's hostility felt personal. Whatever Adam Blackthorn and Judd were hiding, they weren't keen on anyone getting close enough to find out.

As the caravan prepared to set off, Colt approached the head of the line, where Adam Blackthorn was adjusting the reins of his horse. Blackthorn glanced up, his expression guarded, but Colt caught a glimmer of interest in his eyes.

"You're Colt Evans," Blackthorn stated, more as a fact than a question.

Colt nodded. "I heard you were looking for a scout. I'm offering my services."

Blackthorn studied him for a moment, his gaze sharp and calculating. "We're headed into unpredictable territory," he said slowly. "Weather, wild animals, potential raiders... I need someone who can handle whatever comes."

Colt nodded. "I can do that. I've lived off the land most of my life."

Blackthorn's gaze flickered to Judd, who was watching them from a few paces away, his arms crossed. The enforcer's glare made it clear he wasn't thrilled with Colt's addition, but Blackthorn ignored him, turning back to Colt. "Fine," he said, extending a hand. "You're hired. Keep the wagons on track and keep a lookout for trouble."

Colt shook Blackthorn's hand, his grip firm. "You'll have no trouble from me, as long as everyone here stays honest."

Blackthorn raised an eyebrow, a faint smile playing at the corners of his mouth. "Then we understand each other."

With his position secured, Colt took his place at the head of the caravan, his horse's steady gait keeping him slightly ahead of the wagons. His senses remained sharp, his eyes scanning the terrain, but his mind was already focused on his next move. If he stayed close to Blackthorn and Judd, he'd eventually find the answers he was looking for.

As the day wore on, the monotony of the trail was broken only by the occasional murmur of conversation or the sound of horses' hooves against the dirt. Colt noticed Lily Harlow a few wagons back, her posture poised but weary. She kept mostly to herself, occasionally helping an elderly woman or quieting a restless child. Though she was surrounded by others, she seemed distant, as if carrying a weight no one else could see.

In a quiet moment, she glanced up and caught Colt's eye. For a second, he thought she might look away, but instead, she offered a small nod, acknowledging him. Colt returned the gesture, sensing something in her expression—an understanding, perhaps, or the hint of a shared burden.

Toward evening, the caravan came to a halt to make camp. Fires were lit, and the settlers gathered around, sharing stories and hopes for the future. Colt sat a little apart from the others, sharpening his knife by the glow of his own small fire. He was focused on the blade when he sensed someone approaching.

Looking up, he saw Lily standing nearby, her arms crossed against the cool evening air. She hesitated before speaking. "You're the scout now, aren't you?"

Colt nodded, setting his knife aside. "Guess I am. Thought it might be useful, given the folks we're traveling with."

She glanced toward Blackthorn and Judd, who were speaking in low voices at the far end of the camp. "You don't trust them," she said quietly.

Colt shrugged, keeping his voice low. "I trust my own instincts. And they tell me there's more to this journey than Blackthorn's letting on."

Lily seemed to consider this, her gaze distant. "You know, you don't seem like most of the men out here," she said, almost to herself. "Most of them are looking for something—land, gold, a new life. But you... I get the feeling you're running from something."

Her words struck a nerve Colt hadn't expected. For a moment, he considered brushing her off, but there was something about her—a calm resilience that made him feel he could speak the truth, if only a part of it. "I lost someone," he admitted quietly, his voice barely a whisper. "A mentor. He was killed by someone who's somewhere out here on this trail."

Lily's expression softened, and she nodded, understanding lighting her eyes. "Loss does that," she murmured. "It drives people west, looking for peace or revenge."

Colt glanced at her, curiosity piqued. "And what's driving you?"

She held his gaze, a hint of sadness in her eyes. "Someone I lost, too. But maybe, like you, I'm hoping to find answers. Or, at the very least, some peace."

They fell into a comfortable silence, the crackling fire their only witness. Despite their different paths, Colt felt a strange kinship with Lily, a connection that he hadn't felt in years. They both carried their scars quietly, letting the land take some of the weight they couldn't bear alone.

When Lily finally stood to return to her own campfire, she looked back at him, her face softened in the firelight. "Good night, Colt," she said, her voice gentle.

"Good night, Lily."

As she walked away, Colt felt a renewed sense of purpose settle over him. He didn't know where the trail would lead, or what dangers lay ahead, but for the first time, he felt that he wasn't completely alone.

3. Rivers and Rivals

Over the coming weeks, the caravan journeyed deeper into the wild frontier, the sun and moon marking the passage of time across the vast skies. Colt Evans found himself adapting to the rhythm of life on the trail, learning the nuances of guiding the wagons and keeping watch for potential threats. The settlers had slowly begun to rely on him, their trust growing with each mile they traveled and campfire they shared.

The air was crisp as the caravan approached the river that morning, its wide, swift waters rushing ahead, foaming as they collided against stones hidden just beneath the surface. The settlers had grown quiet, each aware of the treacherous crossing that lay ahead. Colt Evans rode at the caravan's head, his gaze sharp as he surveyed the river. The water was high from recent rains, making the crossing riskier than usual, but there was no other route. The trail cut across here, and time wasn't on their side.

As he rode back toward the line of wagons, he noticed Judd Barrett, arms crossed, waiting near one of the front wagons with his usual smirk. Judd had made it clear he wasn't pleased with Colt's position as the scout, but Colt wasn't concerned with Judd's approval. His job was to see this caravan safely to the other side of the river, and no one—especially not Judd—was going to interfere.

"Everyone needs to follow in line," Colt announced, his voice carrying over the sound of the river. "The current's strong. We need to cross in sections, or we risk getting washed away."

Judd scoffed, loud enough for everyone around to hear. "A little water never hurt anyone. You think these folks came all this way just to be scared off by a river?"

Colt felt his muscles tighten, but he kept his tone even. "It's not about fear; it's about safety. We need to keep steady so no one gets swept downstream."

Judd grinned, his eyes narrowing. "Sounds like an excuse for a slowpoke. I say we cross together. Less time wasted on all this worryin'."

The other settlers looked between Colt and Judd, uncertainty flickering in their eyes. Colt could feel the tension thickening around them, the weight of the decision hanging in the air. He took a step forward, meeting Judd's gaze head-on.

"Recklessness will cost lives, Judd. If you want to endanger your own, fine. But you won't be risking these folks," Colt said, his voice low but firm.

Judd's face darkened, his jaw clenched as he took a step closer. For a moment, Colt thought Judd might throw a punch, but instead, Judd's lips curled into a sneer. "You talk a big game for someone new here, Evans. But I don't take orders from you."

Before Colt could respond, a voice broke through the tension. "Is there a problem here?"

Colt turned to see Adam Blackthorn approaching, his face unreadable. The leader's presence seemed to silence Judd, who took a grudging step back. Adam's gaze moved between them, his eyes hard as he waited for an answer.

"Just discussing the best way to cross the river," Colt replied calmly. "I think we should take it slow, one section at a time."

Adam nodded, considering his words. He glanced at Judd, who looked ready to protest, but with a dismissive wave of his hand, Adam silenced him. "Colt's right," he said firmly. "We cross in sections. I won't have anyone risking lives on my watch."

A murmur of agreement passed through the crowd as Adam walked away, and Judd's glare intensified. He leaned in close to Colt, his voice a venomous whisper. "You may have Blackthorn fooled, but I see you for what you are. You're not here to help these people—you're here for yourself."

Colt held Judd's gaze, unfazed. "Believe what you want. But don't expect me to look the other way when you start putting folks in danger."

With a muttered curse, Judd stomped off to the rear of the caravan, and Colt felt a small surge of relief. The other settlers were still watching, but now with trust in his judgment, and Colt was determined not to let them down.

As they began crossing the river, Colt rode ahead, leading the first few wagons in a cautious line. The water was colder than he'd expected, rising nearly to the tops of the wagon wheels, and he could feel the strain in his horse's muscles as they pushed through the strong current. He glanced back over his shoulder to see Lily Harlow among the first group, her eyes steady as she gripped the reins of the mule guiding her wagon.

She caught his glance and gave him a brief nod, an unspoken message of trust that filled him with a rare sense of reassurance. They'd shared a few words the previous night, but he could sense that Lily was beginning to understand his purpose out here, even if she didn't know the full story. Colt could see her admiration growing, even through the veil of wariness that still clouded her gaze.

The crossing was slow and tense, but one by one, each wagon made it to the other side. As the final wagon approached, however, Colt noticed Judd riding alongside it, his face set in defiance. He'd pulled ahead of the wagon line, the wheels dangerously close to slipping out of the narrow path Colt had marked.

"Stay in line, Judd!" Colt called out, his voice hard.

Judd only grinned, his eyes flashing with a challenge. With a kick to his horse's flanks, he surged forward, his horse splashing wildly through the water and sending waves toward the wagon. The driver, a young man barely in his twenties, looked around in panic as his wagon rocked, the wheels slipping off the narrow ledge Colt had scouted.

Without a second thought, Colt spurred his horse forward, charging through the water. He grabbed the horse's reins from Judd's grip, yanking him back just as the wagon tilted dangerously to the side.

"Are you out of your mind?" Colt shouted, barely containing his fury. "You nearly got that boy killed!"

Judd's sneer faltered for a moment, but he quickly masked it with a look of contempt. "I was just showing them how to keep pace. Maybe if you'd done your job right, we wouldn't be wasting time here."

Colt's fists clenched, but he forced himself to take a breath. This was exactly what Judd wanted—to bait him, to make him lose control in front of everyone. "Get back in line," he said through gritted teeth, releasing the reins. "And don't try anything like that again."

Judd muttered something under his breath but relented, guiding his horse back into position. Colt waited until the last wagon had crossed safely, then moved to the rear, keeping a wary eye on Judd. He'd dealt with men like him before, but he couldn't shake the feeling that Judd's recklessness was more than just bravado. There was something else there, a simmering hostility that made Colt's instincts prickle with caution.

As the camp settled down for the evening, Colt took a seat by his small fire, replaying the events of the day in his mind. He was still lost in thought when he felt a presence nearby and looked up to see Lily standing there, her expression unreadable.

"Thank you for what you did today," she said quietly, her eyes meeting his. "I don't think anyone else would've stood up to Judd like that."

Colt shrugged, looking away. "Just doing what needed to be done."

She sat down across from him, studying him with a faint curiosity. "You're a strange one, Colt. You act like you don't care what people think, but then you go out of your way to protect them."

Colt met her gaze, a flicker of vulnerability slipping through his usual guarded expression. "Maybe I see something worth protecting out here," he replied softly. "Folks looking for a new start, trying to build a better life. I'd like to see them make it."

Lily's expression softened, and she smiled, a quiet understanding passing between them. But before either of them could speak, Colt noticed movement at the edge of the camp. Mateo Alvarez, a quiet, sharp-eyed scout, was walking near Adam Blackthorn, his gaze scanning the camp with a calculating glint.

Colt felt a jolt of suspicion. Mateo always seemed to be near Blackthorn, as though watching him, and Colt couldn't shake the feeling that Mateo was more than just a scout. Perhaps he, too, was connected to the death of Colt's mentor, and maybe, just maybe, the answers Colt was seeking lay with him.

As he watched Mateo disappear into the shadows, Colt's resolve hardened. He was close—he could feel it. And soon, he would uncover the truth.

4. The First Attack

Weeks passed by in a blur of dust and toil as the caravan pressed on, traversing harsh terrain and battling the elements. With each passing day, Colt felt the weight of responsibility grow heavier on his shoulders.

The sky bled into shades of deep purple and orange as the sun sank low behind the distant mountains. The camp settled into its usual routine and campfire smoke rose into the cooling night air. Colt Evans sat a short distance from the main cluster of settlers, his senses alert even as he appeared relaxed. Nights like this—when the air seemed almost too still—made him wary.

Lily Harlow was sitting near the fire with a few other women, her gaze occasionally drifting toward Colt. Since the river crossing, she'd found herself watching him more often, though she wasn't quite sure why. There was something about his quiet strength, his guarded but genuine care for the people in the caravan, that pulled her in. But just as she was about to approach him, a sudden rustle from the edge of the camp made her freeze.

Without a word, Colt's hand shot to his rifle, his eyes narrowing as he scanned the darkness beyond the firelight. The murmurs and laughter faded, the settlers sensing something amiss. The silence thickened, charged with a tension that crawled up the spine. Colt stood slowly, his gaze sweeping across the shadowed tree line, his instincts humming with anticipation. Then, a flicker of movement caught his eye.

"Down!" he shouted, diving to the side just as an arrow whistled through the air, embedding itself in the ground where he'd been standing.

Panic erupted. Men and women scrambled for cover as a group of raiders stormed into the camp, their faces painted with dark streaks, their weapons gleaming in the firelight. Shouts echoed as the settlers scattered, many of them too frightened to do anything but hide behind their wagons.

"Colt!" Lily called out, ducking behind a barrel as another arrow sailed past her.

Colt's jaw tightened as he fired a shot at one of the raiders, his eyes never leaving Lily's position. "Stay low!" he shouted, motioning for her to get to the safety of the wagons. He reloaded, his movements quick and efficient, his focus unbroken even as chaos raged around him. He could see Adam Blackthorn a few paces away, standing near his own wagon with his pistol drawn. The guide was barking orders to the few men who were able to gather their wits, but his eyes kept darting nervously to the edges of the camp.

A dark suspicion crept into Colt's mind as he took another shot, dropping a raider who was advancing on one of the settlers. This attack had come almost too suddenly, as if the raiders knew exactly when and where to strike. He clenched his jaw, anger flaring as he took in the terrified faces of the settlers around him.

"Everyone, behind the wagons!" he called out. "Form a line, keep your backs to the fires. They're using the shadows to get close!"

Slowly, the settlers rallied, following Colt's orders as he moved through the camp, picking off raiders one by one with calculated shots. Judd Barrett, who had been lounging by his own fire earlier, finally charged forward, a pistol in each hand as he took down a couple of the attackers with impressive precision. Despite his earlier disdain for Colt, Judd seemed to recognize the gravity of the situation, his face set in a grim determination.

"Nice of you to join us, Judd," Colt muttered, firing off another shot as Judd passed by.

"Don't flatter yourself, Evans," Judd snarled, but there was no malice in his voice this time, only focus as he fired into the dark.

With Colt and Judd leading the defense, the settlers began to push back against the raiders. Gradually, the attackers faltered, their numbers thinning as Colt's relentless fire forced them to retreat. The remaining few melted into the darkness, leaving behind only the silence and the soft crackling of the campfires.

Breathing heavily, Colt lowered his rifle, his gaze sweeping across the camp to ensure everyone was safe. The settlers emerged from their hiding places, their faces a mixture of relief and admiration as they looked to Colt. His steady presence had kept them from breaking, had turned what could have been a massacre into a victory.

Lily hurried over to him, her face pale but determined. "Are you hurt?" she asked, her voice quiet but filled with concern.

Colt shook his head, giving her a reassuring nod. "I'm fine. You all right?"

She nodded, managing a small smile. "Thanks to you."

Colt felt a warmth settle in his chest at her words, though he forced himself to look away, not wanting her to see how much her gratitude meant to him. "Just doing what needed to be done," he said gruffly, his tone neutral even as he fought to steady his pulse.

But his relief was short-lived. The suspicion that had been gnawing at him since the start of the attack resurfaced, sharper now, and he turned his attention to Adam Blackthorn, who was talking in hushed tones with Mateo Alvarez. Colt watched them closely, noting the tension in Adam's posture, the wary glance he cast toward Colt.

Colt made his way over, his steps measured, his face unreadable. When he reached Adam, the other man looked up, a guarded expression in his eyes. Mateo stepped back, his expression carefully blank.

"Trouble finding our way through the forest?" Colt asked casually, his gaze steady on Adam. "Those raiders knew exactly where to hit us. Almost as if someone led them right to us."

Adam's eyes narrowed slightly, a flicker of irritation passing over his face. "What are you implying, Evans?"

Colt held his gaze, his voice low. "Just seems strange, that's all. Raids like this don't usually happen without someone tipping them off. I just hope our guide isn't hiding something that could get us all killed."

Adam's face hardened, but he forced a smile. "You think I'd risk my own life along with everyone else's, Evans? That's a bold accusation to make without proof."

Colt shrugged, his eyes unwavering. "Proof or no proof, I don't trust coincidences out here. Too many lives are at stake."

Adam's forced smile slipped, his face tightening with barely concealed anger. "I don't know what you're after, Evans, but if you're looking for trouble, you'll find it." With that, he turned sharply and walked away, Mateo trailing after him, casting a wary glance over his shoulder.

Colt watched them go, his suspicions only deepening. He'd seen the look in Adam's eyes before—the look of a man hiding something, desperate to keep it buried. Colt couldn't shake the feeling that Adam was more involved in this ambush than he'd ever admit, and the nagging thought of his mentor's murder gnawed at the edges of his mind. Was Adam connected to that, too?

As Colt moved back toward the camp, he felt someone fall in step beside him. It was Lily, her face shadowed with worry as she kept pace with him.

"What was that about?" she asked softly, her eyes searching his face.

Colt sighed, glancing away. "Nothing that'll sit easy," he replied. "I think there's more to Blackthorn than he lets on."

Lily looked back toward where Adam had disappeared, her brow furrowing. "You really think he's involved?"

"I don't know," Colt admitted, his voice low. "But I aim to find out."

Lily nodded, her gaze steady. "You're not alone in this, Colt. I'm here to help however I can."

Colt met her gaze, feeling a surge of gratitude he hadn't expected. For years, he'd been a lone wolf, relying on no one but himself. But now, with Lily beside him, he felt something shift—a sense of companionship he hadn't realized he was missing.

"Thank you, Lily," he said quietly, the sincerity in his tone surprising even him. She gave him a small smile, her hand brushing his arm in a gesture of reassurance.

As the night deepened the camp settled into an uneasy rest. Colt took up his position on watch, his senses honed. Experience told him it would be a long night, but he was sure they'd safely see the sunrise.

5. Storm on the Plains

The caravan endured not only the challenges of the trail but also the weather of the plains. Rain lashed at the canvas tents, and the winds howled like a living beast. Colt was learning that the frontier was unforgiving, demanding resilience from those who dared to tread its path. Each day brought new struggles, but Colt remained a steadfast presence.

Threaening clouds loomed over the horizon, swelling like a coiled serpent ready to strike. The smell of rain hung heavy in the air, a warning sign that the fierce storm rolling across the plains was fast approaching. The once-clear skies had turned ominous, and Colt Evans could feel the tension in the caravan as unease rippled through the settlers.

"Gather up the livestock! Get the wagons close together!" Colt shouted, his voice cutting through the rising wind. He moved swiftly among the pioneers, urging them into action as the first drops of rain began to fall, each one a cold reminder of the storm's fury.

As the winds picked up, Lily Harlow rushed over, her face set with determination. "What do we need to do?" she asked, her hair whipping around her face.

"We have to make sure the wagons are secure and that everyone is ready to move if we have to," Colt replied, scanning the camp for any signs of danger. "We can't let this storm catch us off guard."

Behind them, Judd Barrett leaned against a wagon, arms crossed and a smirk plastered on his face as the rain began to pour. "What a sight, huh?" he called out mockingly, his voice barely audible over the wind. "I thought we were tougher than this. Maybe some of you city folk don't belong out here."

Colt turned, anger flaring in his chest. "Shut it, Judd. This isn't the time for your nonsense."

"Oh, but it is," Judd replied, his tone dripping with contempt. "You think you're the only one who knows how to handle a storm? This is what separates the wheat from the chaff. I say let it pour. Maybe some of these softies will finally learn a lesson."

Colt stepped forward, ready to confront Judd, but Adam Blackthorn arrived just in time, his expression grim. "We're all in this together, Judd.

Enough with the theatrics. We need to make sure everyone is accounted for."

Judd's smirk faltered, but he quickly masked it, shrugging off Adam's words. "Sure, but it's not my fault if they can't handle a little rain."

Ignoring Judd, Colt moved through the chaos, directing the settlers to work together as the winds howled, and the rain began to lash down in earnest. He felt the pressure of their trust building as they looked to him for guidance. In moments like this, every small action mattered.

With each wagon secured and the livestock rounded up, the storm unleashed its full fury. Thunder boomed overhead, and lightning crackled across the sky, illuminating the scene with blinding flashes. The winds howled, threatening to tear through the camp, and Colt shouted to the settlers, urging them to find shelter.

"Get to the wagons! Stay low! Hold on to anything you can!" he yelled, his voice straining against the elements. The settlers scrambled, fear evident in their eyes, but Colt remained focused, guiding them with steady authority.

In the midst of the chaos, he spotted Lily again, struggling against the wind as she tried to secure a tarp over one of the wagons. He rushed over, grabbing one end of the tarp and helping her to secure it against the onslaught of rain.

"Thank you!" she shouted, her eyes bright with determination, even as the storm threatened to drown them out. "I don't know how we'd manage without you!"

Colt felt a surge of pride at her words, even as he fought against the downpour. "Just doin' what I can," he replied, trying to keep his tone light, though he could feel the weight of the storm pressing in around them. "We need to stick together. That's the only way we'll make it through."

As they worked side by side, the energy between them shifted, a silent understanding forming amidst the chaos. Colt could see the strength in her, the resolve to push forward despite the storm. But there were shadows in her eyes, doubts she hadn't spoken yet, and he wondered if they could weather not just the storm but the challenges that lay ahead.

Just then, a bolt of lightning struck a nearby tree, splintering it with a deafening crack that sent everyone screaming and diving for cover. The raiders were forgotten, the earlier conflict eclipsed by the sheer power of nature, and Colt felt the pulse of adrenaline coursing through him.

"Stick together! Don't scatter!" he shouted as the wind roared around them, shaking the very ground beneath their feet. The caravan was their home, their lifeline, and they needed to protect it at all costs.

After what felt like hours, the storm finally began to abate. The rain turned from a torrential downpour to a steady drizzle, the winds calming as the skies began to clear. Colt looked around, surveying the damage. A few wagons were toppled, but thankfully, no one had been seriously hurt.

Lily brushed rain-soaked hair from her face, a mixture of relief and exhaustion visible in her eyes. "I can't believe we made it," she said, her voice low.

Colt took a deep breath, shaking the water from his hair. "We did, but it wasn't easy. You all did great."

A faint smile broke through her expression, a spark of admiration igniting in her gaze. "You were amazing, Colt. I don't know how you stay so calm in the middle of all that."

Colt shrugged, the praise making him feel uncomfortable yet appreciated. "Just keepin' my head, I guess. Someone has to lead."

"But it's more than that," Lily insisted, her voice firm. "You inspire everyone. You make them feel safe." She paused, her eyes searching his. "And you've inspired me, too."

Colt felt a flush of warmth at her words, but he was careful to keep his expression neutral. "I'm just doing what needs to be done," he repeated, the familiar wall rising between them. "We all have our roles."

"But what about your role?" Lily pressed, stepping closer, her expression earnest. "What do you want for yourself, Colt? This is a chance for all of us to start over, to find a new path."

He hesitated, the weight of her question settling heavily on his shoulders. "I want to make sure you all get where you're going safely," he said, but even to him, the answer felt inadequate.

"And then what?" she asked softly. "What happens when we reach our destination?"

Colt glanced away, the storm having exposed more than just the elements outside. "I don't know," he admitted, his voice barely above a whisper. "I'm just a trapper. I've always been on my own."

Lily's expression shifted, her vulnerability surfacing. "But you don't have to be alone anymore. We could help each other, Colt. We could make a life here."

As much as her words stirred something deep within him, Colt couldn't allow himself to entertain such thoughts. He'd spent too long focused on revenge, on finding the men who had taken everything from him. Letting someone in could lead to complications he wasn't ready for.

"I have my own path," he finally said, his voice steady. "And right now, it's about getting you and the rest of the caravan to safety. That's all that matters."

Lily's gaze dropped, disappointment flashing across her features, but Colt couldn't bear to see it. He turned away, his heart heavy with a mix of emotions he couldn't quite articulate. He had no right to drag her into his troubles, to let her get close when he was still lost in his own darkness.

The aftermath of the storm left the caravan in disarray, but Colt focused on the task at hand. They needed to regroup, to make repairs, and he wasn't about to let Judd or Adam take advantage of the situation.

As the settlers began to clear debris and set things right, Colt spotted Adam moving toward him, his expression unreadable. Colt braced himself, feeling the tension between them linger in the air like an unspoken challenge.

"Nice job out there," Adam said, though his tone was clipped. "You managed to keep everyone alive."

"Thanks, but we still have a long way to go," Colt replied, keeping his voice steady. "You should be doing more than just standing around, Blackthorn."

Adam's eyes narrowed, and for a moment, they stood toe-to-toe, the weight of their unspoken conflict hanging between them. Colt could feel the energy crackling, both men unwilling to back down, each one holding a thread of doubt about the other.

"I lead this caravan," Adam replied coolly, his posture rigid. "You might have impressed some folks today, but I'm still in charge here. Just remember that."

Colt felt a flash of irritation at the challenge in Adam's voice, but he nodded, refusing to let his emotions flare. "We all need to do our part if we want to survive out here. I'm just trying to help."

Adam's expression softened for a moment, and Colt could see the flicker of uncertainty in his eyes. "We all have our secrets, Colt. Just be careful how you tread."

As Adam walked away, Colt felt the weight of his words pressing down on him. He had questions swirling in his mind, doubts that refused to settle. The storm may have passed, but the clouds were far from gone. He needed to stay vigilant, to protect those who depended on him, and to uncover the truth before it was too late.

6. An Uneasy Alliance

The mood was tense as the caravan moved forward. The settlers were weary, both from the storm and the uncertainty that hung over them. Supplies were dwindling, and their destination still lay far beyond the horizon. Colt Evans felt the pressure mounting—not just on him, but on everyone. They needed to reach safety soon, or desperation would set in.

Colt had been observing Mateo Alvarez more closely since the storm. The cunning scout had always had a presence about him, a shifty demeanor that made Colt wary. But in this situation, Colt knew he might need Mateo's sharp instincts if he were to expose Adam Blackthorn's intentions. The last confrontation between Adam and Colt had only deepened the divide, and Colt couldn't shake the feeling that

Adam was hiding something critical about the caravan's future.

The two men finally crossed paths one evening by the river, where the settlers had gathered to refill their supplies. Colt leaned against a tree, arms crossed, his eyes scanning the horizon as the last remnants of the day's light faded. The sound of rushing water filled the air, a calming rhythm that was almost at odds with the tension that crackled between him and Mateo.

"Evans," Mateo said, approaching with a wary smile. "Seems like you've been doing a lot of watching lately."

Colt narrowed his eyes. "And you've been lurking. What do you want, Mateo?"

Mateo chuckled, but there was a hint of nervousness in his demeanor. "Just trying to survive, same as you. But I can't help but notice you're not exactly on good terms with our esteemed guide."

Colt straightened, shifting his weight. "Let's cut to the chase. I need your help. I suspect Adam knows more about the raiders than he's letting on."

Mateo raised an eyebrow, leaning against a nearby rock as if trying to gauge Colt's sincerity. "You think so? Adam's been around the block a few times. He knows how to survive out here."

"Yeah? Well, so do I," Colt snapped. "But I don't set people up to take a fall. If you've got any information, I need you to share it. We can't afford to trust him blindly."

Mateo sighed, rubbing his chin thoughtfully. "You know, I've always been good at reading people. You're passionate about this, I'll give you that. But Adam has his own reasons for keeping things close to the vest. He's not just some brute; he's a survivor."

Colt stepped closer, lowering his voice. "And you're a survivor, too. You've been in enough tough spots to know when someone's playing games. What's your angle, Mateo?"

A flicker of uncertainty crossed Mateo's face. "Let's say I'm caught in the middle. Adam trusts me, but I see the way you've rallied the others. You could be a leader, Colt, if you wanted. But I'm not sure I can betray Adam without knowing what's at stake for him."

"Your loyalty is to the people in this caravan, not to Adam," Colt insisted, frustration building. "If you want a shot at redemption, help me uncover the truth. We're running out of time."

Mateo regarded him for a long moment, the silence stretching between them. "You think you can expose Adam? And what happens then? If you're right, he could retaliate. He has a reputation, Colt."

Colt clenched his fists, feeling the weight of the moment. "I'm not afraid of Adam. What I'm afraid of is losing everyone in this caravan to whatever games he's playing. Help me figure it out, and we'll find a way to keep everyone safe."

Mateo's expression shifted, a hint of respect shining through. "You're a bold man, I'll give you that. Alright, I'll keep my ears open. But you need to understand—I'm not choosing sides yet. I have my own agenda."

"Just remember that we're in this together," Colt replied, feeling a flicker of hope. If Mateo had his ear to the ground, it could be invaluable.

As they spoke, a loud commotion erupted from the camp, pulling their attention away. Colt and Mateo hurried back, finding Judd Barrett standing over Lily, his face twisted into a menacing grin. The air around them crackled with tension as Judd leaned closer, looming over her.

"What's this, Harlow?" he taunted, his voice dripping with disdain. "Thought I told you to keep your distance from the trapper. He's nothing but trouble, and you'd do well to remember that."

Lily stood her ground, though her expression was tight with fear. "I can make my own choices, Judd. Colt's just trying to help."

"Help? Or lead you right into danger?" Judd scoffed, taking a step closer. "You're too good for a life like this, and you're letting that fool drag you down."

Colt felt his blood boil, stepping forward to shield Lily. "Back off, Judd. You don't get to threaten her."

Judd's eyes narrowed, and for a moment, it seemed as if the entire camp held its breath. The settlers had gathered, their faces reflecting a mix of fear and anticipation. Colt could see them watching, waiting to see how the confrontation would unfold.

"Or what?" Judd growled, his voice low and dangerous. "You think you can stand up to me? You think you're some sort of hero?"

Colt took a deep breath, steadying himself. "I don't need to be a hero, Judd. I just need to protect the people who matter."

The tension thickened, and for a heartbeat, it felt as if the world was about to explode around them. Then Judd straightened, a cruel smile creeping onto his face. "You're a fool, Evans. But I'll give you this—you've got guts. Just know that in this world, guts don't keep you alive."

With that, Judd turned and sauntered away, leaving Colt and Lily standing there, the air still crackling with unspoken tension. Colt felt a surge of anger, the adrenaline of the confrontation still coursing through him.

"Are you alright?" he asked Lily, concern etched across his features.

She nodded, though her eyes were wide, reflecting the fear she had tried to hide. "I'm fine. Judd just... he's always like that."

"Yeah, well, it's not going to fly with me," Colt said, his tone fierce. "No one's going to push you around, Lily. Not while I'm here."

Her expression softened, gratitude shining through the fear. "Thank you, Colt. You've done so much for all of us."

"I just want to make sure everyone is safe," he replied, but the words felt hollow in his chest. Beneath the gratitude was a truth they both knew: the dangers they faced weren't just from the outside, but also from within.

Later that night, as the stars struggled to peek through the remaining clouds, Colt sat by the fire, his thoughts swirling. Mateo had agreed to help him, but he couldn't shake the feeling that the scout had his own motives. Trust was a luxury he couldn't afford, but with supplies dwindling and Judd growing more aggressive, they needed all the allies they could muster.

With a sigh, Colt glanced toward the wagon where Lily was resting. She had been a beacon of hope in the chaos, and yet, the weight of his own secrets loomed heavy. He couldn't allow himself to get too close. Not now. He had a mission to fulfill, a promise to keep, and distractions could cost them everything.

The night grew colder, the fire crackling as he stoked the flames, but as he stared into the flickering light, Colt felt a sense of determination solidifying within him. He would protect the caravan, uncover the truth behind Adam's intentions, and perhaps, just perhaps, find a way to keep the ghosts of his past from dragging him down.

7. The Crossing

The caravan had made considerable progress, the rolling plains finally giving way to rugged terrain. As the settlers neared the treacherous mountain pass a tension hung heavy over the group. Colt Evans could feel it in his bones—this part of the journey would test their resolve like never before.

The path ahead twisted and turned, steep cliffs looming on one side while a steep drop-off bordered the other. It was the kind of place that could lead to disaster if not navigated correctly. Colt took a deep breath, the scent of pine and earth grounding him momentarily. But as he approached the front of the caravan, he spotted Adam Blackthorn surveying the mountain pass with an unsettling calm.

"We're taking this route," Adam declared, his voice steady yet authoritative. "It'll save us time and lead us to the river before the snow starts falling."

Colt's stomach churned. "That's not a good idea, Adam. The trail is narrow and unstable. We could easily lose wagons or worse—lives."

Adam turned, annoyance flashing in his eyes. "And what do you suggest, Evans? We detour and waste precious time? The longer we linger out here, the more danger we invite."

Colt stepped forward, raising his voice to carry over the murmurs of the settlers, many of whom had gathered to listen. "We've already faced enough peril on this journey. A reckless decision like this could cost us everything. We should take the safer route."

A ripple of agreement spread through the crowd, and Colt felt the weight of their support bolster his resolve. He scanned their faces, seeing the fear and uncertainty reflected back at him. They were desperate for a leader, someone who could steer them away from danger.

Adam's expression darkened. "You think you can sway these people with your bravado? They need a guide, not a doubter. I've led countless expeditions through these mountains. I know what I'm doing."

Colt's heart raced, and he stepped closer, challenging Adam's authority. "But at what cost? You're more interested in saving time than ensuring their safety. This isn't just a journey; it's their lives on the line."

Mateo, having heard the commotion, stepped forward, his expression contemplative. "Colt makes a point, Adam. We've seen what happens when we rush without caution. Maybe it's worth considering a safer path, even if it takes longer."

A murmur of agreement rippled through the settlers, emboldening Colt. He could feel the tide shifting, and he pressed on. "We can't afford to gamble with our lives. This isn't just about reaching our destination; it's about making sure we get there together."

"Enough!" Adam roared, his voice echoing off the mountains, silencing the crowd. "You're trying to incite rebellion among the settlers, Colt. You want to lead? Then you better be prepared to take responsibility for everyone's safety. Otherwise, stand down and let me do my job."

Colt clenched his jaw, but the fear in the settlers' eyes pushed him onward. "I won't stand down while you make decisions that could endanger us all. If we have to choose between speed and safety, I vote for safety!"

"Let's vote!" a voice cried out from the back of the crowd. It was a man Colt recognized from their travels—a farmer, weary but resolute.

The call for a vote resonated through the group, gathering momentum. The settlers were frightened, but they also wanted a voice in their fate. Colt seized the opportunity. "Everyone who agrees that we should take the safer route, raise your hands!"

One by one, hands went up, hesitant at first but then with growing confidence. Colt's heart raced as he counted, the numbers climbing higher, and the realization dawned on Adam that he was losing control. The settlers were looking to Colt for guidance, and he couldn't let them down.

Adam's face turned a deep shade of crimson, rage simmering beneath the surface. "This is insubordination," he hissed, but the murmurs of the crowd drowned him out.

"Safety over speed!" Colt called, his voice strong and unwavering. "We have families here, children, lives. If we're to survive this journey, we have to do it together and smartly!"

As the vote concluded, it became evident that the settlers overwhelmingly favored Colt's suggestion. Adam's fury was palpable, and Colt braced himself for the storm that was about to unfold.

"Fine," Adam spat, his voice low and menacing. "We'll take the safer route. But mark my words, Evans, you've just cost us valuable time. You're going to regret this."

Colt met his gaze, unflinching. "Maybe you'll see that this isn't just about you, Adam. It's about the people we're supposed to protect."

With a scowl, Adam turned on his heel, storming off into the shadows of the trees. Judd Barrett followed closely behind, his eyes narrowing in thought. Colt knew the confrontation hadn't ended; it had only begun.

As dusk settled over the mountains, the caravan began to make preparations for the safer route. Though Colt felt a rush of victory, he couldn't shake the feeling that Adam would retaliate.

Judd's demeanor had grown increasingly hostile, and Colt sensed danger lurking just out of sight.

"Colt!" Lily called out, rushing to his side as they worked together to secure the wagons for the new path. Her eyes sparkled with admiration. "You did it! You stood up to him."

"It was a team effort," he replied, grateful for her support but keenly aware of the challenges ahead. "But we're not out of the woods yet. Adam and Judd won't take this lightly."

"I know," she admitted, her brow furrowing in concern. "They seem… dangerous."

"They are," Colt said, scanning the horizon where Adam and Judd had disappeared. "But we have to stay strong. This caravan needs leadership, and if it's going to be me, then I need everyone's trust."

Lily placed a reassuring hand on his arm. "You have mine, Colt. And I think you have theirs, too. We can face whatever comes next, as long as we do it together."

The warmth of her touch sent a spark of determination through him, and he nodded, taking a deep breath. "Right. Together. We'll get through this."

As the caravan set out on the safer route, Colt felt a renewed sense of purpose. They had chosen the path of caution, but he knew it was just the beginning of their struggles. Behind the scenes, Adam and Judd were plotting, and he had to be ready for whatever they would unleash.

Night fell, wrapping the mountains in darkness, but the flickering campfires cast long shadows, reflecting the uncertainty that lay ahead. Colt knew the danger wasn't just from the elements or the mountains; it came from within their own ranks. And as long as Adam and Judd were around, they would stop at nothing to regain control.

8. Secrets Revealed

Colt Evans sat near the fire, lost in thought, his mind racing with the implications of Adam Blackthorn's recent defiance. The decision to take the safer route had earned him the respect of the settlers, but he knew the storm wasn't over. Adam and Judd would be plotting their next move.

Just then, Mateo Alvarez approached him, his expression serious and unreadable. Colt recognized the weight of urgency in Mateo's demeanor and felt a shiver of apprehension. "Colt, can we talk?" Mateo asked, glancing around as if checking for eavesdroppers.

Colt nodded, motioning for Mateo to join him further from the firelight. "What's on your mind?"

Mateo hesitated, then took a deep breath. "There's something I've been meaning to tell you—something important about your mentor."

Colt's heart raced at the mention of his mentor. "What do you know? What happened to him?"

Mateo looked around again before continuing, his voice barely above a whisper. "I knew him well, Colt. He was a good man, and he didn't deserve what happened. Adam... he was involved in it. Your mentor was looking into something that Adam didn't want exposed."

Colt's breath caught in his throat. "What do you mean? What was he investigating?"

Mateo clenched his fists, anger flashing across his face. "Your mentor suspected Adam of running illicit trades through the caravan routes—dealing with raiders and corrupting innocent settlers. He was gathering evidence when he disappeared. I didn't want to believe it, but the pieces fit together."

"Illicit trades?" Colt repeated, disbelief and fury warring within him. "Adam is a murderer?"

"I can't say for certain that he pulled the trigger," Mateo replied, anguish etching lines across his brow, "but he was definitely involved. And Judd? He's been his enforcer for years. They'll do anything to protect their interests."

Colt felt the rage bubbling beneath the surface, and a wave of determination surged through him. "We have to expose them. The settlers need to know the truth."

"I want to help you," Mateo said, his voice firm now. "But we need to gather evidence first. If we confront them without proof, they'll turn the settlers against us."

Colt nodded, his mind racing with possibilities. "We can't let Adam get away with this. If he's willing to kill for his secrets, who knows what else he's capable of? But we need to act quickly. If they realize we're onto them, it could put everyone in danger."

Just then, a familiar voice cut through the tension. "What's going on?" It was Lily, her expression curious and concerned. She had approached quietly, her keen intuition guiding her toward their hushed conversation.

"Lily!" Colt said, surprised. "We were just discussing—"

But Mateo interrupted, his gaze locked on Lily. "You shouldn't be here. It's dangerous."

"Dangerous?" she challenged, crossing her arms defiantly. "What's dangerous is not knowing what's happening in our own caravan. Colt, I want to help. I can't just stand by while you face this alone."

Colt exchanged a glance with Mateo, who looked torn. "This is bigger than all of us, Lily," Colt said, lowering his voice. "If we expose Adam and Judd, we risk everything."

"I know that," she replied, her voice steady. "But I can't sit back and let you carry this burden alone. I've seen how they treat the settlers. They're bullies, and it's time we stand up to them. I want to help you gather evidence, Colt."

Colt felt a surge of warmth at her determination. "Alright. But we have to be careful. Adam and Judd are smart and ruthless. If they catch wind of what we're planning..."

Lily nodded, her expression resolute. "We'll be careful. But we can't let fear dictate our actions. Together, we can do this."

Mateo studied Lily for a moment before nodding slowly. "If we're going to move forward, we need a plan. We should start gathering any evidence we can find against Adam. He may have left a trail, something we can use to convince the settlers."

Colt's heart raced with a mix of hope and trepidation. "Alright. Here's what we'll do. We'll start by talking to the settlers—see if anyone has noticed anything strange. I'll keep an eye on

Adam and Judd, and we need to watch for any interactions that might reveal their true motives."

Lily smiled, her eyes sparkling with determination. "I can talk to the women in the caravan. They might have seen or heard something that we haven't."

Colt felt a sense of unity forming, a bond strengthened by a shared purpose. "Let's meet back here after dark. If we can uncover anything concrete, we'll decide on our next steps."

As the trio dispersed into the night, Colt's mind raced with thoughts of what lay ahead. The mountain pass loomed behind them, a reminder of the treacherous journey they faced. But now, with Lily and Mateo at his side, he felt a flicker of hope.

Hours later, as the fire crackled low and the moon cast a silver glow over the camp, the three reconvened. Colt sat cross-legged on the ground, his heart pounding with anticipation as Lily and Mateo shared what they had discovered.

"I spoke with some of the women," Lily began, her voice filled with excitement. "They mentioned that supplies had gone missing during the last few days—food, ammunition, even some personal belongings. No one knows where it went, but it's suspicious, especially with Judd keeping watch."

Mateo nodded, his expression thoughtful. "That could be a sign that Adam and Judd are up to something. If they're diverting resources to fund their schemes, it could tie into what happened to your mentor."

Colt felt a rush of adrenaline, a sense that they were closing in on something vital. "If we can gather enough evidence about the missing supplies, we might be able to confront them directly. But we need to keep our eyes peeled for anything else they might be doing."

Just then, a loud shout pierced the night air, causing all three of them to freeze. "What now?" Colt whispered, his heart racing.

"Sounds like trouble," Mateo said, peering into the darkness beyond the campfire.

Before they could react, a group of settlers rushed toward them, panic etched across their faces. "It's Adam and Judd!" one of them shouted, breathless with fear. "They're gathering the men—they're plotting something!"

Colt's pulse quickened. "What do you mean? What are they planning?"

"They're angry about the vote," another settler replied, his voice shaky. "They think you're trying to take control. They want to teach you a lesson."

Colt exchanged glances with Lily and Mateo, his heart sinking. They were running out of time. "We need to warn the others and prepare for a confrontation. If they think they can intimidate us, they're dead wrong."

Colt rallied the settlers. The truth about Adam and Judd was surfacing, and he would stop at nothing to protect those who had placed their trust in him.

Together, they would stand strong, and Colt vowed that he would not allow Adam's treachery to go unpunished. The mountain pass loomed ahead, but they would navigate its challenges together, armed with the truth and the courage to fight for their freedom.

9. Final Confrontation

The caravan moved cautiously through the winding paths of the mountain pass. Adam Blackthorn's deception had been laid bare, and Colt was determined to face him head-on.

As they pressed deeper into the mountains, Colt sensed that Adam was up to something. He had grown increasingly agitated, his eyes darting around as if searching for an escape route. Colt's instincts screamed at him that Adam was leading them to an isolated location, one where he could eliminate Colt and flee without a trace.

"Stay close," Colt warned the settlers, his voice low but firm. "We need to watch each other's backs. I have a feeling Adam is planning something desperate."

Lily Harlow stood beside him, her expression fierce and resolute. "We'll protect each other, Colt. Whatever Adam has in mind, we'll be ready for it."

As they approached a clearing surrounded by steep cliffs, Colt's heart sank. This was the place Adam had chosen—a dead end with no easy escape. The settlers slowed their pace, sensing the impending confrontation. Colt's instincts were on high alert, and he glanced at Mateo, who stood vigilant near the back of the caravan.

"Get ready," Colt whispered, drawing his rifle closer. "We need to be prepared for anything."

Suddenly, Adam's voice rang out, cutting through the tension like a knife. "Stop! This is where it ends, Colt. You've meddled long enough!"

Colt's breath caught in his throat as Adam emerged from the shadows, flanked by Judd Barrett. The brutish enforcer stood menacingly at Adam's side, his fists clenched and ready for a fight. The settlers exchanged fearful glances, and Colt could see the fear reflected in their eyes.

"Adam, it's over," Colt said, stepping forward, his rifle trained on Adam. "We know what you did. You've betrayed these people, and now you're going to pay for it."

Adam's lips curled into a cold smile. "You think you've won, don't you? But you're wrong. You're just a thorn in my side, and I'll cut you out. Judd, take care of him."

Before Colt could react, Judd lunged forward, a primal roar escaping his lips. Colt barely had time to react as the brute barreled toward him, fists swinging. He sidestepped just in time, feeling the wind of Judd's punch rush past him. The fight was on.

"Get back!" Colt shouted to the settlers as he engaged Judd, dodging another powerful blow. The mountain echoed with the sounds of fists striking flesh, the grunts of exertion filling the air.

Colt ducked low, narrowly avoiding a blow that could have knocked him off his feet. "Lily!" he shouted, spotting her nearby. "Get the others to safety!"

But Lily stood her ground, eyes blazing with determination. "I'm not leaving you!" she cried, her hands balled into fists. "We fight together!"

"Damn it, Lily!" Colt growled, but before he could argue further, Judd charged at him again. Colt pivoted, delivering a swift kick that sent Judd stumbling back.

In that moment of chaos, Lily spotted an opportunity. Judd was momentarily off balance, and she seized the chance to distract him. "Hey, Judd! Over here!" she shouted, waving her arms to catch his attention.

Judd turned, confusion flashing across his face. "What are you doing?" he roared, but Lily's boldness had given Colt the opening he needed.

With adrenaline surging through him, Colt lunged at Judd, landing a solid punch to his jaw. The enforcer staggered, and Colt pressed his advantage, throwing a flurry of punches that sent Judd reeling.

"Keep fighting, Colt!" Lily shouted, her voice fierce and unyielding. "We can't let them win!"

Adam watched the chaos unfold, his expression shifting from confident to panicked as he realized that his plans were unraveling. "Judd! Get up! We need to end this!"

As Colt grappled with Judd, he felt the brute's massive strength pushing him back. Colt used every ounce of his strength, leveraging his agility against Judd's brute force. He ducked low, sweeping Judd's feet out from under him. The enforcer hit the ground hard, gasping for breath.

Colt turned his attention to Adam, who was now frantically searching for an escape route. "It's time to face the music, Adam," Colt said, advancing on him. "You've caused enough pain. You can't run anymore."

Adam's eyes darted around, calculating his next move. "You think you can take me on alone?" he sneered, backing away. "You have no idea who you're dealing with."

"Then let's find out," Colt said, his grip tightening on his rifle. "You're not just a murderer—you're a coward hiding behind others. It ends here."

Adam's bravado wavered as he glanced back at Judd, who was slowly recovering, groaning as he pushed himself off the ground. Colt felt the tide of the confrontation shifting in his favor, but they weren't out of the woods yet.

With a fierce shout, Judd charged at Colt again, but this time, Colt was ready. He sidestepped and swung his rifle, catching Judd in the side of the head. The impact sent the enforcer sprawling back to the ground, unconscious.

Lily took advantage of the distraction, darting toward Colt. "What now? We need to finish this!" she urged, her eyes fierce with determination.

"Help me keep Adam contained," Colt replied, glancing at the remaining settlers, who were watching the chaos unfold with wide eyes. "If we can restrain him, we can expose his treachery to everyone."

With newfound resolve, Colt and Lily approached Adam together, flanking him as he backed away, desperation etched on his face.

"You're making a mistake," Adam warned, his voice trembling. "You have no idea who I am!"

Colt stepped forward, refusing to back down. "You're a liar and a coward, hiding behind your enforcer. You think you can control us? You're wrong. We'll fight for our lives, and we'll make sure everyone knows the truth."

Adam glanced at the other settlers, who had begun to close in, emboldened by Colt's stand. The fear in Adam's eyes deepened, and he knew he was cornered. "You'll regret this," he spat, but his bravado was hollow, revealing the cracks in his facade.

With a sudden movement, Adam reached for a hidden knife at his belt, but Colt was faster. In one swift motion, he lunged forward and knocked the knife from Adam's grip. It clattered to the ground, far out of reach.

"You've lost, Adam," Colt said, breathing heavily as he stared down the man who had caused so much pain. "It's time to answer for your crimes."

Lily stepped forward, determination burning in her eyes. "We'll make sure everyone knows what you've done. Your days of hiding are over."

Colt's heart raced as he surveyed the scene. The settlers stood behind him, united in their resolve. Adam, now stripped of his power and bravado, looked around, panic written across his face.

"Don't think this is over," Adam hissed, a tremor in his voice. "You think you can take me down? You don't know the kind of people I'm connected to!"

Colt shook his head, steeling his resolve. "We're not afraid of you anymore. You've lost your hold over us."

With that, the settlers surged forward, encircling Adam and ensuring that he could no longer escape. Colt felt the weight of their collective strength, a force that would no longer be manipulated or bullied.

As Adam's face twisted in fury and desperation, Colt finally felt a sense of closure wash over him. The fight was hard-won, but he had stood against the darkness and emerged victorious. This journey had been about survival, but it had also been about reclaiming their freedom.

With Lily at his side, Colt turned to face the horizon. They had faced down the dangers together, and now it was time to embrace the dawn. Together, they would build a new life free from the shadows of the past, ready to face whatever challenges lay ahead.

10. New Beginnings

The sun rose over the rugged mountains to mark a new day, bathing the world in a warm golden light that seemed to chase away the shadows of the past. Colt Evans stood at the edge of the camp, his heart lighter than it had been in years. The air carried with it the scent of pine and the promise of new beginnings.

Adam Blackthorn and Judd Barrett were restrained in a wagon, ready to be handed over to the first lawman or army outpost they came upon. The settlers began to pack up. Colt felt a swell of pride at the sight of them—ordinary men and women transformed into a fierce, united community. They had faced darkness together and emerged stronger.

"Colt!" Lily called, her voice bright and buoyant. He turned to see her striding toward him, her hair catching the sunlight like a halo. She was a beacon of hope in a world that had often felt dark and unforgiving.

"Morning," he replied, smiling as she approached. "How are the others holding up?"

"They're ready to move," she said, her eyes sparkling with excitement. "It's a new day, and I think they can feel it too. There's a sense of relief in the air."

Colt nodded, glancing back at the camp where the settlers were gathering their belongings. "After everything we've been through, it feels good to finally have a chance to breathe. I still can't believe how far we've come."

Lily stepped closer, her gaze steady. "You did more than just lead them, Colt. You fought for them. You brought them together when it seemed like everything was falling apart."

Colt felt warmth wash over him at her words. "I couldn't have done it without you, Lily. You were my anchor when everything felt overwhelming."

A soft blush crept across her cheeks, and she looked away, a shy smile playing on her lips. "We make a good team, don't we?"

"Yeah, we do," Colt said, his heart swelling with emotion. In that moment, he realized how deeply his feelings for her had grown. It was no longer just about admiration or gratitude; it was something much deeper, a connection forged through shared trials and triumphs.

As the settlers finished their preparations, Colt felt a sudden pang of loss as he thought about the road ahead. "We have a long way to go, don't we?" he said, glancing toward the distant horizon.

"We do," Lily replied, her voice steady. "But it's a journey we'll make together. And this time, we can choose our destination."

Colt took a deep breath, feeling the weight of his past slowly lift from his shoulders. The thirst for revenge that had fueled him for so long was gone. He realized that seeking vengeance would only continue the cycle of pain. Instead, he wanted to build something meaningful, something that would honor the memory of his mentor while also creating a brighter future.

"Adam and Judd may have tried to destroy us," Colt said, his voice filled with conviction. "But we're not defined by what they did. We have a chance to create something better—a place where people can thrive and feel safe."

Lily smiled, her eyes shining with hope. "A community built on trust and compassion. That's what we can do."

As the caravan began to move, Colt felt a excitement bubble within him. Each creak of the wagon wheels and rustle of the horses' reins signaled a new chapter in their lives. He looked over at the settlers, their faces reflecting determination and resilience.

"Let's make this journey count," Colt called out to the group, his voice strong and steady. "We have the chance to build something incredible, and I want each of you to know that your voices matter. We'll work together to create a future we can all be proud of."

Cheers erupted from the settlers, their spirits lifted by Colt's words.

As they made their way down the trail, Colt felt a gentle touch on his arm. He turned to see Lily gazing at him, her expression soft. "Colt, I—"

But before she could finish, a loud shout echoed from the back of the caravan. "Look out!" One of the settlers had spotted something in the distance, and Colt's heart raced as he scanned the horizon.

"What is it?" he asked, instinctively reaching for his rifle.

Lily's eyes narrowed as she squinted into the sun. "I don't know, but it looks like a group of riders."

The settlers fell silent, fear creeping into their expressions. Colt stepped forward, determination flooding his veins. "Stay close to the wagons. I'll see what's happening."

He moved swiftly, taking charge of the situation. As he approached the edge of the clearing, he raised his rifle, prepared to defend his newfound family. But as the riders came closer, Colt's heart sank in disbelief.

"Wait!" one of the riders called out, waving a white flag. Colt recognized the man immediately—his old friend and fellow trapper, Jack Turner.

"Jack! What are you doing here?" Colt shouted, lowering his rifle.

Jack rode up, dismounting quickly. "We heard about what happened up here. We came to help."

The tension in Colt's chest eased as relief washed over him. "We've had our share of trouble, but it's finally over. Adam and Judd won't be a threat anymore."

Jack's eyes widened, and he nodded. "Good. We wanted to join you on this journey. There are others who are ready to stand with you."

Colt felt a surge of hope at Jack's words. The caravan was growing, and with it, the possibilities for a new beginning. "Join us," he said, motioning for Jack to bring his group forward. "We could use more hands. Together, we can build something that lasts."

As Jack called for his companions to join them, Colt felt Lily's presence beside him, her hand brushing against his. "See? You're already creating the community you dreamed of," she said softly, pride lighting up her features.

Colt turned to her, a smile spreading across his face. "This is just the beginning, isn't it?"

Lily nodded, her eyes reflecting the golden light of the rising sun. "We have a long road ahead, but I believe in what we can create together."

As the caravan continued down the trail, Colt felt a profound sense of peace wash over him. The journey had transformed him, and though the path had been fraught with danger and uncertainty, he had emerged with a renewed spirit.

He glanced around at the settlers—people who had once been strangers, now united by a common purpose. He felt a warmth in his heart as he realized that he had found not only a community but also a partner in Lily, someone who shared his vision for a better future.

Together, they would forge a new life in the uncharted lands ahead, their hearts filled with hope and determination. Colt knew that the trail of redemption lay before them, a path illuminated by the promise of new beginnings. He was ready to embrace whatever awaited them, knowing that with each step, they were writing their own story—one of resilience, love, and an unbreakable bond forged in the fires of adversity.

Other Books from Seniorality

To find your next book visit:
www.amazon.com/author/seniorality
Where you will find:

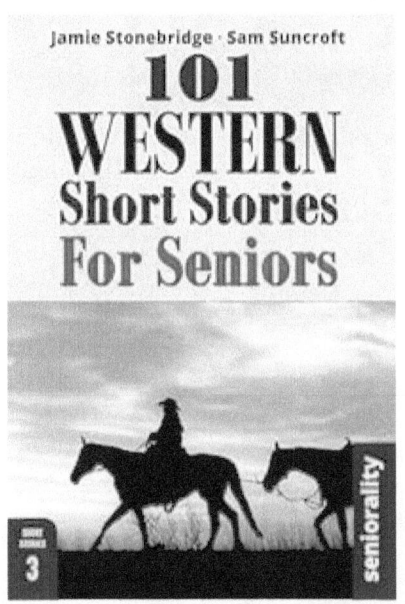 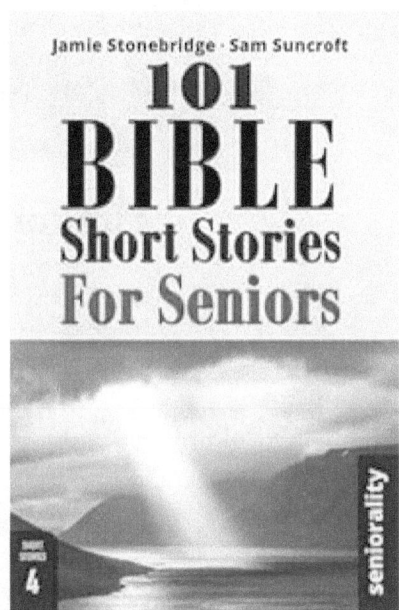

Short Stories

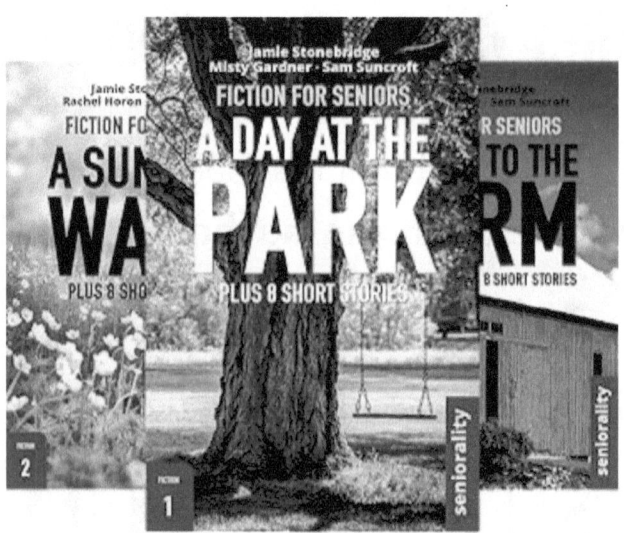

Fiction for Seniors

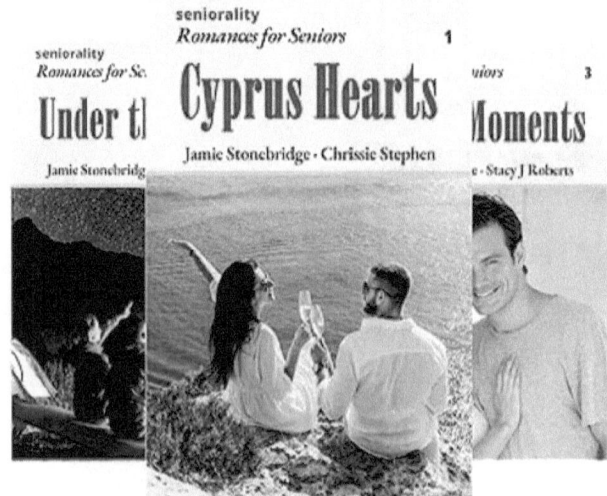

Romances for Seniors

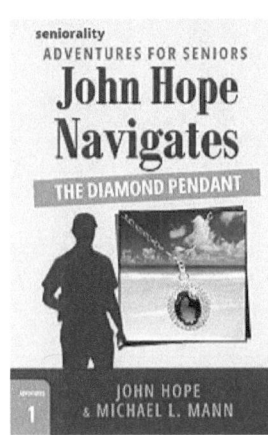 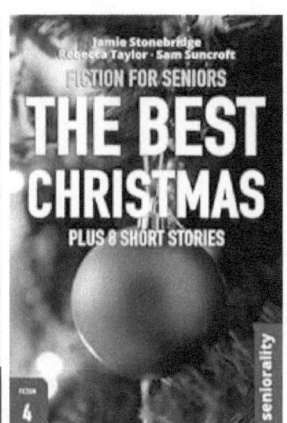 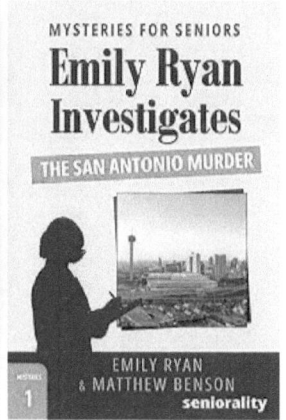

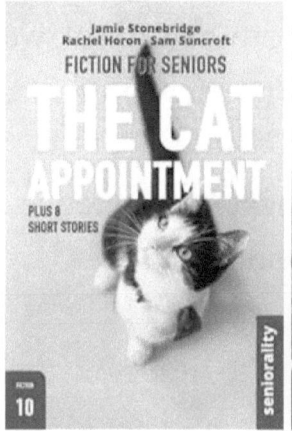 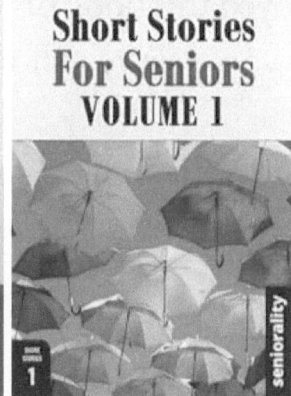

And More

Find these books by searching on Amazon for
'seniorality'

or visit:

www.amazon.com/author/seniorality

Thank You

If you enjoyed this book or found it useful, we'd be very grateful if you'd write a short review on Amazon.

Your support really does make a difference and helps other people discover this book.

We personally read all reviews to hear how the books are being used, to collect feedback, and get ideas for future stories.

Thank you and have a wonderful day!

www.ingramcontent.com/pod-product-compliance
Lightning Source LLC
Chambersburg PA
CBHW020439220526
45464CB00002B/778